Understanding Obesity: A New Hope For Weight Loss and Escaping Food Addiction

Copyright Notice

No part of this book may be reproduced or transmitted in any form whatsoever, electronic, or mechanical, including photocopying, recording, or by any information storage or retrieval system without expressed written, dated and signed permission from the author. All copyrights are reserved.

Disclaimer

Reasonable care has been taken to ensure that the information presented in this book is accurate. However, the reader should understand that the information provided does not constitute legal, medical or professional advice of any kind.

No Liability: this product is supplied "as is" and without warranties. All warranties, express or implied, are hereby disclaimed. Use of this product constitutes acceptance of the "No Liability" policy. If you do not agree with this policy, you are not permitted to use or distribute this product.

We shall not be liable for any losses or damages whatsoever (including, without limitation, consequential loss or damage) directly or indirectly arising from the use of this product.

Claim This Now

<u>Autoimmune Healing Transform Your Health, Reduce Inflammation, Heal the Immune System and Start Living Healthy</u>

Do you have an overall sense of not feeling your best, but it has been going on so long that it's actually normal to you?

If you answered yes to any of these question, you may have an autoimmune disease.

Autoimmune diseases are one of the ten leading causes of death for women in all age groups and they affect nearly 25 million Americans.

In fact millions of people worldwide suffer from autoimmunity whether they know it or not.

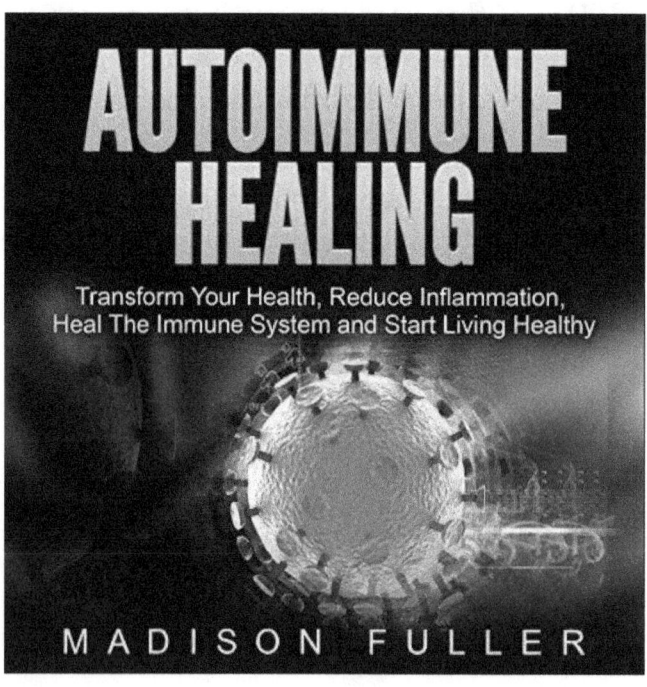

Want More?

Sign up to get the exclusive Madison Fuller e-newsletter, sent out a few times a week:

Sign Up

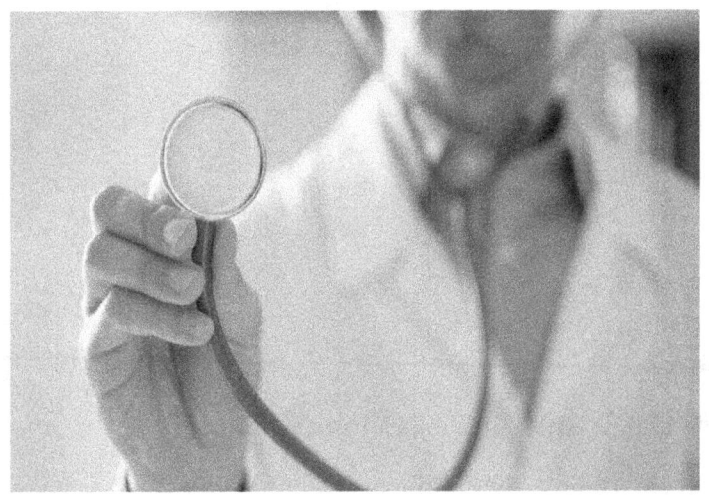

Table of Contents

Introduction

Chapter 1 Obesity Explained
- Genetic factors
- Over-eating
- Sedentary lifestyle
- Medication
- Psychological factors
- Diseases
- Social issues

Other Factors associated with Obesity
- Ethnicity
- Childhood weight
- Hormones
    - Insulin
    - Sex hormones
    - Growth hormones
    - Inflammatory factors
- Behavioural factors

Chapter 2 Symptoms of Obesity

Steps in the diagnosis of Obesity
- Health history
- General physical exam
- Calculating BMI
- Measuring the circumference of the waist
- Checking for other health issues
- Blood tests

Screening for Obesity
- Underwater weighing
- BOD/POD
- DEXA

Skin calipers
　　Bioelectric impedance analysis (BIA)
　　Weight-for-height tables in determining Obesity

Chapter 3 Risks of Obesity
　　Insulin resistance
　　Type 2 diabetes
　　High blood pressure
　　Heart Disease
　　Stroke
　　Cancer
　　Sleep apnea
　　Osteoarthritis
　　Fatty Liver Disease
　　Kidney disease
　　Pregnancy problems

Chapter 4 Macronutrients and Micronutrients
　　Macronutrients
　　Micronutrients

Chapter 5 Portion control
　　Reducing Binge Eating
　　Glucose Level Balance
　　Bolstering Satiety
　　Weight Loss or Maintaining a Healthy Weight

Chapter 6 Obesity Myths
　　Myth 1- Genes are to Blame for Obesity
　　Myth 2 - Lack of Self-Control is Responsible for Obesity
　　Myth 3 - The Obesity Epidemic is driven by a Lack of Access to Fresh Vegetables and Fruits
　　Myth 4 - It is not overeating that Causes Obesity, but it is leading a too Sedentary Lifestyle
　　Myth 5 – Better Education Regarding Diet and Nutrition can help in Conquering Obesity
　　Myth 6 – Carbohydrates are Bad, Get Rid of them from the Diet

Chapter 7 Role of Diet

Role of medication in the treatment of obesity
    Phentermine
    Orlistat

Role of weight loss surgery in the treatment of obesity

Are meal substitutes, artificial sweeteners, and over-the-counter (OTC) products effective in treating obesity?
    Meal substitutes
    Artificial Sweeteners
    Over-the-counter weight-loss products

Chapter 8 Healthy Eating Plan
    Weight regulation
    Increase productivity
    Save money on life insurance
    Enhance mood
    Be healthier

Foods: The Good and Bad
    Avocados
    Eggs
    Beans
    Yogurt
    Salmon
    Fruits
    Almonds

Healthy Eating Tips

Conclusion

Have you been thinking of shedding off some of your fat? Are you interested in healthy body weight?

Well, the answer to these questions often varies from one individual to another. However, the most important thing is for you to know what healthy body weight is for you. Obesity is something that goes beyond just a cosmetic concern! You have to realize that obesity can take a toll on your body and place you at risk of serious diseases like heart disease, type 2 diabetes, some cancers, and hypertension, among others. Most of these diseases stem from several underlying metabolic abnormalities that often affect the muscle, liver, pancreas, and other tissues in the body.

According to statistics, more than half of the American population are obese, and what is even more shocking is that about 60% of this population are children and adolescents. However, the good news is that there are various strategies you can employ in losing weight and taking control of your body weight. Just bear in mind that weight-loss is a long-term journey that begins with a single step!

Most of the treatment guidelines recommend that people who are obese should aim to lose at least 5-10% of their initial weight during the first month of their weight-loss program if they are going to attain their goals. Additionally, these treatments are much more successful when they are used in combination with dietary changes and regular exercises.

In this book, you will learn;

- The risk factors of obesity

- The importance of portion control
- Obesity and hormones
- Debunking the myths about obesity
- Role of diet, medication, and surgery in the treatment of obesity
- Whether meal substitutes, artificial sweeteners, and over-the-counter (OTC) products are effective in treating obesity
- The good and bad foods
- Tips for healthy eating

So, what are you still waiting for? Come with me and let's delve deeper into understanding obesity and how to shed off that extra pound for a healthy body!

Introduction

Did you know that obesity is one of the biggest health concerns in the world? Well, the truth is, statistics show that obesity has tripled since 1975. According to research conducted in 2016, over 1.9 billion adults were found to be overweight. Out of these, over 650 million were obese. What is even shocking is that more than 41 millions of this obese population are children under the age of 5 and 340 million are children and adolescents between 5 and 19 years.

One thing that we have to realize is that most of the world's population reside in countries where obesity kills. Obesity is, in fact, a condition often associated with a large number of health conditions collectively referred to as metabolic syndrome. Some of these conditions include; high blood sugar levels, elevated blood pressure as well as poor blood lipid profiles, among others. Such people with metabolic syndrome are at a higher risk of developing heart disease as well as type 2 diabetes as compared to those with normal body weight.

In the last few decades, there has been so much research directed on understanding obesity and finding ways to prevent or treat it. The good news is that obesity can be prevented. Many people think that obesity is brought about by a lack of willpower. Although weight gain is often a result of our eating habits and lifestyle, some people are at a disadvantage as far as controlled eating is concerned.

Overeating is something that is controlled by a wide range of biological factors such as genetics and hormones. There are those who are predisposed to weight gain. You may be thinking that people can overcome their genetic disadvantage, and you are right because this requires a shift in lifestyle and behaviour. However, these require one to have strong willpower, perseverance, and a triple dose of dedication.

Nevertheless, claiming that behaviour is something that is purely a function of willpower is being overly-simplistic, mainly because they fail to consider other factors that ultimately have a role to play in determining what people do and when they do it.

The good news is that even when one is obese, they can still lose a modest amount of weight and improve their health. This is something that can be achieved through proper dietary changes, improved physical activities, as well as behavioural changes that favour weight loss. You can also achieve this using various medications and weight loss surgery. However, you have to ensure that you seek the advice of your health professional to know which option works best for your condition.

After all, is said, you have to understand that maintaining ideal body weight is a matter of balancing the consumption of food and calories required by the body for energy. In other words, you have to think of it in the sense that you are defined by what you eat. It is the types and amounts of food you eat that influences your ability to maintain ideal body weight and weight loss. U.S. Department of Agriculture has put in place various dietary guidelines like;

- Consumption of a variety of foods
- Balancing between the food you eat with plenty of physical activities
- Selecting a diet with a variety of fruits, grains and grain products
- Selecting diets that are low in cholesterol, fats and saturated fats
- Selecting diets that have moderate amounts of sugars
- Selecting a diet that has a moderate amount of salt and sodium
- Finally, if you are used to taking alcoholic beverages, you do so in moderation

Chapter 1 Obesity Explained

Let us just say that the definition of obesity often varies based on what you read. Generally, you can think of obesity and being overweight as having a weight greater than what is recommended as a healthy weight. Additionally, obesity refers to a chronic condition that is characterized by an excess amount of fats in the body. The truth is, a certain amount of body fat is necessary for storage of energy, shock absorption, and heat insulation, among others.

To better define obesity, we can think of it in terms of body mass index (BMI). In other words, the body mass index is equivalent to a person's weight (kilograms) divided by their height (square meters). Because BMI describes the body weight relative to height is an indication of a strong correlation with total body fat in an adult. For an adult, a BMI of between 25 and 29.9 is termed as being overweight, and anything above 30 is termed as obese. If you have normal body weight, your BMI should be between 18.5 and 24.9. However, if your BMI is something above 40, then this is termed as morbidly obese.

It is important that you understand that there has to be a balance between your caloric intake and the amount of energy your body uses, hence determining what your weight is. If you consume lots of calories than you burn, you are likely to put on more weight since the body will store up the excess in the form of body fats. On the contrary, if you eat fewer amounts of calories than you metabolize, you are likely to lose weight. Therefore, one of the most common causes of obesity is brought about by overeating and lack of physical exercise. Ultimately, the body weight is determined by metabolic, genetic, behavioral, environmental, and cultural factors.

Genetic factors

If your parents are obese, there is a high chance that you will develop obesity as well. One important thing that you have to note is that genetic factors often affect hormones that play a role in fat regulation. For instance, one of the genetic causes of obesity is the deficiency of leptin. Leptin is a hormone produced by fat cells and the placental cells. This hormone plays a central role in the control of weight by simply signaling the brain to consume less whenever the levels of body fats in storage are way too high.

However, if for one reason or another the body is not able to synthesize adequate amounts of leptin or that leptin is not able to send a signal to the brain to consume less, the control is lost and hence promoting the occurrence of obesity. Currently, researchers are exploring the role of leptin replacement as an obesity treatment option.

Over-eating

If you often overeat diet that is high in fat, there is a chance that you will put on more weight. One thing that people fail to realize is that foods that are high in fats and sugars possess a high energy density, hence contributing to weight gain.

Additionally, if you overeat diets that are high in simple carbohydrates, there is a high chance that you will put on more weight. Carbohydrates are high in sugar levels, and this increases blood glucose levels. This, in turn, stimulates the release of insulin from the pancreas. Insulin plays a central role in promoting the growth of fat tissues, hence contributing to weight gain.

Other research scientists believe that certain simple sugar foods like wine, soft drinks, desserts, and beer contribute so much to weight gain. This is because they are easily absorbed into the blood stream compared to complex carbohydrates like grains, raw fruits, brown rice, pasta, and certain vegetables. Because of this, they cause an increase in the release of insulin soon after meal intake. The higher the amount of insulin in the blood, the higher the chances of weight gain.

Frequency of eating is another form of overeating. One thing that is not well understood is how the frequency of eating and weight gain are related. According to certain studies, there are reports of people who are overweight eating less often compared to those with normal body weight. Those who eat small meals often (4-5 times a day) appear to have lower levels of cholesterol. This means that they have more stable blood sugar levels compared to those who eat less frequently (2-3 meals). The possible explanation for this is that when you take small meals frequently, your insulin levels are more stabilized, while large meals cause a large spike in insulin soon after meals.

Sedentary lifestyle

It is interesting that although people know the importance of physical activity in weight loss and maintaining healthy body weight, they still lead a sedentary lifestyle. Some examples of a sedentary lifestyle include;

- Sitting in an office without much physical movement
- Playing computer games for prolonged hours without engaging in physical activities
- Using your car to run errands throughout without considering the option of taking a walk or cycling

These are just but a few examples of sedentary lifestyles. One thing that you have to bear in mind is that the lesser you move around physically, the fewer the calories you burn, hence contributing to weight gain.

Additionally, you have to realize that the lesser you engage in physical activities, the more your hormonal activity is affected, and you know hormones influence how the body processes food. So many studies have demonstrated that physical activity goes a long way in keeping the insulin levels much stable, hence keeping your weight in check. Even though certain research study designs make it quite difficult to draw inferences accurately, incorporating regular exercises into your lifestyle plays a key role in maintaining as well as boosting several aspects of your overall health, including sensitivity to insulin.

You do not have to be training in a gym for you to be physically active. You can take part in so many physical activities, walking, household chores, going up and down the stairs, cycling, among others. However, what you have to realize is that the intensity and type of activity you choose affects the degree to which it is beneficial to the body both in the short- and long-term.

Medication

There are so many medications that are associated with weight gain and ultimately causing obesity. Some of these medications include; anticonvulsants, diabetes medications, antidepressants, hormonal medications like oral contraceptives, and several corticosteroids. Additionally, certain high blood pressure medications and antihistamines may contribute to weight gain and obesity.

The reason why these medications promote weight gain varies from one medication to the other. If you have a concern over this, it is critical that you s=discuss with your physician other alternative options instead of discounting the entire medication on the accounts of weight gain and obesity, without necessarily looking at the serious effects this might have on your health condition.

Psychological factors

For certain people, their emotional well-being may influence their eating habit. For instance, if you are sad, stressed, angry, or bored, you may be prone to turn to food as an escape. While so many people who are overweight or obese lack psychological disturbances compared to normal weight people, over 30% of people seeking obesity treatment often experience trouble with binge eating.

Diseases

There are several diseases like hypothyroidism, Cushing's syndrome, insulin resistance, and polycystic ovary syndrome, among others that predisposes one to obesity.

Social issues

According to research, there is a strong link between obesity and social issues. For instance, if you lack money to buy healthy foods or live in a place that has no secure walking paths or places to exercise, then there is an increased risk of becoming obese.

Other Factors associated with Obesity

Ethnicity

It has been shown that ethnicity factors can influence one's age of onset as well as the rapidity of weight gain. African-American and Hispanic women tend to put on more weight early in life compared to Asians and Caucasians. On the other hand, Hispanic and Hispanic black men have a high rate of obesity compared to non-Hispanic white men. However, the prevalence is significantly lower in men than in women.

Childhood weight

According to certain studies, your weight during childhood, teenage years, and early adulthood has so much to do with the possibility of developing obesity during adulthood. For instance, if you were mildly overweight during your early 20's, there is a high chance that you might be obese by the age of 35. If you were overweight during older childhood, this could be predictive of obesity in adulthood, especially if you have a genetic predisposition to obesity. Finally, if you are overweight during your teenage years, there is a high chance that you will be obese in adulthood.

Hormones

During certain hormonal linked events, there is a high chance that one might gain weight. In women, this can be during pregnancy, menopause, among others like the use of contraceptives. However, with the advent of contraceptive pills that are lower in estrogen, weight gain is no longer a great risk factor.

Hormones are often referred to as chemical messengers that play a key role in regulating various body processes. They are one of the factors that contribute to obesity. Such hormones as leptin (discussed earlier), insulin, sex hormones, as well as growth hormones often influence metabolism, appetite, and distribution of body fats. Obese people have certain levels of these hormones that promote abnormal metabolism and subsequent accumulation of body fats.

It is the role of the endocrine system to secrete hormones into our bloodstream. Additionally, the endocrine, nervous, and immune systems work together hand in hand to help the body cope with certain stresses. When there is an excess of certain hormones or a deficit of others, this can promote the occurrence of obesity.

1. *Insulin*

Insulin is a hormone that that is secreted by the pancreas, and it plays a central role in regulating carbohydrate and fat metabolism. It is the work of insulin to stimulate the uptake of glucose from the blood in such tissues as the muscles. This is a process that is very critical in ensuring that energy is available for proper functioning and maintenance of normal glucose levels in circulation.

For someone that is obese, the most unfortunate thing is that the insulin signals are lost and hence, the body tissues are no longer able to control the levels of glucose. Therefore, this can lead to type 2 diabetes as well as metabolic syndrome.

2. *Sex hormones*

The distribution of body fats is important in the development of obesity-related diseases like stroke, heart disease, arthritis, among others. If fats accumulate around the abdomen, this poses a greater risk for diseases compared to when they accumulate around such regions as the hips, bottom, and thighs. According to research, there is evidence that demonstrates the role of androgen and estrogen in the distribution of body fats. Oestrogen is a sex hormone that is secreted by the ovaries in women during the pre-menopausal stage to promote ovulation.

However, some men and women do not produce enough estrogen from their testicles and ovaries, respectively. Rather, lots of these sex hormones are produced in body fats, even though they are in lower quantities. In younger men, the androgen is produced in high quantities, and the levels reduce as they grow older.

This change in the levels of sex hormones with age often results from changes in the distribution of body fats. While women of childbearing age store their body fats on the lower parts of their body, older men and women in their menopause increase the level of fat storage around their abdominal region. Additionally, women who are on estrogen supplements do not accumulate fats on their abdomens. Some animal experiments demonstrate evidence of excessive weight gain whenever there is a lack of estrogen.

3. *Growth hormones*

It is the role of the pituitary gland in the brain to secrete growth hormone. This is the hormone that plays a role in determining one's height and hence helps build their bone and muscle structure. The growth hormone also affects the rate of metabolism. In other words, people who are obese tend to have lower levels of growth hormones compared to those with a normal weight.

4. *Inflammatory factors*

It is important to note that obesity is often associated with chronic inflammation within the fat tissues. Whenever there is excessive storage of fats, there are stress reactions in the fat cells that in turn, promotes the release of proinflammatory factors from the fat cells as well as immune cells in the adipose tissue.

Behavioural factors

Did you know that obese people have certain levels of hormones that promote the accumulation of body fat? Certain behaviours like overeating and physical inactivity cause a reset of processes that are critical in regulating appetite and distribution of body fats. This renders one to be physiologically susceptible to weight gain. The truth is, the body is constantly looking for ways to maintain balance, hence resisting short-term disruptions like crash dieting.

When one ingests a low-calorie diet, the blood levels of leptin reduces. It is these lower levels of leptin that plays a key role in increasing one's appetite and slows down the rate of metabolism. This explains the reason why such people engage in crash diets hence regaining the energy that they had initially lost. Leptin therapy may someday be able to help such people.

Nevertheless, evidence of long-term behavioural changes offers an opportunity for one to retrain their bodies to shed off excess pounds and keep it off. It is also evident that weight loss is a result of adopting a healthy diet plan, surgery, and exercise, which leads to improved insulin resistance, modulation of obesity hormones, and reduced inflammation. It is also important to note that weight loss is associated with a low risk of developing heart diseases, some cancers, type 2 diabetes and stroke, among others.

Chapter 2 Symptoms of Obesity

One of the first warning signs that you are overweight is if your body weight is above average and your calculated BMI is 27 and above. Therefore, if you are obese, you may start seeing the following;

- A large body weight
- Excessive fat accumulation on your upper arms, thighs, and waist
- An unproportioned facial structure like having a double chin
- Skin problems mainly brought about by moisture accumulating around skin folds
- Sleep apnea
- Breathing problems
- Lethargy
- Varicose veins
- Gallstones
- Whiteish and purplish patches around the abdomen
- Osteoarthritis

Steps in the diagnosis of Obesity

If you have a BMI that is way above 30, then you know that you are obese. It is the responsibility of your physician to take details of your health history before they can perform any physical exam and recommend tests.

Here are some of the exams and tests that are used in the diagnosis of obesity;

1. Health history

The very first thing that the doctor is required to do is review your health history, weight history, eating habits, weight-loss efforts, exercise habits, among others. They also should know your history of medications, levels of stress, and whether you have had any other issues about your health. It is also important that they know your family history to determine whether you have predisposing factors to obesity.

2. General physical exam

This involves taking measurements of the patient's height, weight, and vital signs like temperature, heart rate, and blood pressure, among others. You may also have to listen to the heart and the lungs as well as examining the abdomen.

3. Calculating BMI

It is important to measure the patient's Body mass index to determine whether they are obese or not. This is an exam that is recommended to be done annually. It is this BMI that plays a significant role in determining your overall health risk as well as what treatment or medication is suitable for your condition.

4. Measuring the circumference of the waist

The fat that is stored around the waist region is often referred to as the abdominal or visceral fat. It is the accumulation of fats around this region that increases one's risk of developing heart diseases and diabetes. According to research, women with a waist circumference of greater than 35 inches have a higher health risk compared to people with smaller waist circumference. Just like your BMI, it is also important that you measure your waist circumference at least once a year.

5. Checking for other health issues

If there are diseases or health problems that you know you have, it is important that your Physician knows so that they can evaluate them. It is also important that the doctor checks for other possible health risks that you may not know of like diabetes and hypertension.

6. Blood tests

The tests your doctor recommends often depends on your overall health after the exam as well as related risk factors that you may have. Some of the common blood tests may include fasting glucose, cholesterol test, thyroid test, and liver function test, among others. The doctor might also recommend that you have an electrocardiogram to check the state of your heart.

All this information goes a long way in helping the physician determine how much weight you need to lose as well as the health risks you already have. All these will play a role in guiding the treatment plan.

Screening for Obesity

There are so many methods that you can employ when measuring obesity. One thing you have to bear in mind is that measuring one's percentage of body fats is not easy and, in most cases,, is prone to inaccuracy if care is not taken into consideration when performing it. Some of the methods you can use include the following;

Underwater weighing

This is also referred to as hydrostatic weighing. This method works by weighing a person under water and then calculating their lean body mass and body fat. It is one of the most accurate methods. However, the only downside is that it is quite expensive.

BOD/POD

This is a computerized method that looks like an egg-shaped chamber. It employs a similar principle to the hydrostatic weighing method mentioned above. However, it measures the mass and volume and uses that in determining the whole-body density. Using this kind of data, you can then calculate the body fat and the lean muscle mass.

DEXA

This is referred to as Dual-energy X-ray absorptiometry. It measures the density of the bone. Using the X rays, it can determine both the body fat percentage as well as the amount of fat found in the body.

Skin calipers

This is a simple and straightforward method that you can use to measure the skinfold thickness of the fat layers under the skin. You can do this for various parts of the body. You then use the results obtained to calculate the percentage of body fat.

Bioelectric impedance analysis (BIA)

This technique is composed of two methods. One of the methods involves using footpads to stand on a custom scale. A small, non-harmful amount of electric current is sent into the body so that body fat percentage is calculated.

The other type of BIA uses electrodes that are placed on the wrist and the right hand as well as the foot. Voltage changes between the two electrodes is measured and used in calculating the percentage of body fat.

That said, so many health clubs, as well as weight-loss centers, use the skin calipers or bioelectric impedance analysis methods. However, you have to note that they are prone to giving inaccurate results if performed by someone who is not well trained/inexperienced. They also are prone to inaccuracies when used on someone with significant obesity.

Weight-for-height tables in determining Obesity

One of the methods used in determining whether one is obese is the weight-for-height tables. While each measurement method has its shortcomings, they serve as reasonable indicators that the subject being measured has a problem with their weight. The good thing with this method is the fact that calculations are quite easy, and you do not need any special equipment to determine obesity.

In spite, the fact that this method is so old (developed in 1943), the Metropolitan Life insurance company introduced their tables based on policyholders' data so that they could easily relate their weight to disease and mortality rate. Doctors have widely used these tables in determining whether their patient is overweight or not. This is mainly because these tables have a range of weights that are acceptable for a person of a certain height.

One of the shortcomings of these tables is the fact that there is no agreement among doctors on one universal table to use. Each one believes in a different version with varying weight ranges. Some consider one's frame size, sex, and age, while others do not.

That said, one of the most significant limitations is the fact that these tables are not able to distinguish between muscle and fat. In other words, someone muscular may be considered obese based on the table readings, when they are, in fact, not obese.

Chapter 3 Risks of Obesity

One thing that you have to bear in mind is that obesity is not just a cosmetic condition, but also harmful to your overall health. This is because it serves as a risk factor to so many diseases mentioned briefly in the section above. In the U.S. alone, over 112,000 people die annually because of obesity, whether directly or indirectly. Most of these deaths are people with a BMI of greater than 30. What is important to note is that people who are morbidly obese (i.e., BMI >40) have a generally reduced life span.

Some of the risk factors of obesity include;

Insulin resistance

As mentioned earlier, insulin is a hormone that plays a central role in the transportation of blood glucose into muscle cells and fats. Transportation into cells plays a critical role in helping insulin keep the levels of blood glucose in the normal range. So, what is insulin resistance?

Well, insulin resistance refers to a condition where there is low effectiveness of insulin in the transport of glucose into the cells. Fat cells appear to have high insulin resistance compared to muscle cells. Therefore, the main cause of insulin resistance is obesity. What is interesting is that, in response to insulin resistance, the pancreas produces more insulin.

As the pancreas continues to produce sufficient amounts of insulin to counter the resistance, the blood sugar levels are kept at normal levels. The insulin resistance state can last for several years. As soon as the pancreas is no longer able to keep up with high production of insulin, the blood sugar levels start going up, hence leading to type 2 diabetes. Hence, insulin resistance can be termed as a pre-diabetes condition.

Type 2 diabetes

It is important to note that the extent and duration of diabetes increase the risk of type 2 diabetes. Type 2 diabetes is highly linked to central diabetes. In other words, someone with central diabetes is one that has excess amounts of fats around their waist region.

High blood pressure

The other risk factor of obesity is hypertension. According to a Norwegian study, there is evidence that shows that weight gain increases with increased blood pressure in women much more than in men.

Each time your heart beats, blood is pumped through the arteries to the entire body. However, hypertension has no symptoms but is likely to cause serious conditions like stroke and heart disease. Normal blood pressure is said to be 120/80 mm Hg. However, if the number at the top is higher than 140 and the lower one higher than 90, then you are said to be hypertensive.

Having a large body weight increases one's risk of developing high blood pressure. This is mainly because the heart is required to pump blood harder to supply all other cells in the body. Excessive fats also cause damage to the kidneys that are responsible for blood pressure regulation.

Heart Disease

This is a term that is often used to describe various conditions that affect that heart. One of the most common problems is that associated with the thickening and narrowing of blood vessels, hence reducing the amount of blood and oxygen supplied to the heart. If you have heart disease, there is a high chance that you will experience heart failure, angina, heart attack, and abnormal heart rhythms, among others. This is one of the leading causes of death in the U.S.

If you are obese, this increases your risk of developing heart disease with such health issues as high blood pressure, high blood sugar, and high blood cholesterol. Additionally, having an excess weight often makes it quite challenging to pump blood to various cells in the body. It is therefore important that you aim at losing weight to improve pressure, flow, and cholesterol levels.

Stroke

When the blood flow to the brain is stopped, the brain cells die and hence leading to stroke. One of the most common types of stroke is an ischemic stroke that occurs when a blood clot blocks the artery that supplies blood to the brain. The other type is referred to as hemorrhagic stroke that occurs when the blood vessels in the brain suddenly burst.

People who are obese or overweight often induce an increase in blood pressure, which is the leading causes of stroke. To reduce the risk of stroke, it is critical that you ensure that your blood pressure is under control. If you lose weight, you may be able to lower the blood pressure, improve blood cholesterol and sugar, hence lowering the overall risk of stroke.

Cancer

This often occurs when the cells in one part of the body are abnormally proliferating. The cancerous cells then begin to spread to other parts of the body like the liver, hence is the second leading killer disease in the U.S.

Obesity has been shown to increase the risk of developing several types of cancers like breast cancer, colon/rectum cancer, gallbladder cancers, and kidney cancers, among others. The mechanism by which this happens is still not well understood. However, what is clear is that cancer cells use glucose as their main source of nutrients and energy. Therefore, adopting a ketogenic diet, exercising regularly, and adopting a healthy diet can contribute to weight loss and reduced risk of cancers.

Sleep apnea

This refers to a condition in which an individual experiences one or more breathing pauses during sleep. This brings about daytime sleepiness, difficulty paying attention and in extreme cases may lead to heart failure.

One of the most important risk factors of sleep apnea is obesity. Someone who is obese may have excess fats stored around the neck region, causing the airways to become smaller, hence promoting difficulty in breathing or snoring. Breathing may also stop altogether for short durations.

Additionally, excess fat stored around the neck region has been shown to produce certain substances that promote inflammations. If the inflammation occurs around the neck, this often leads to sleep apnea.

Osteoarthritis

This is a very common health issue that causes joint pains and stiffness. It is often related to an injury or aging and in most cases affects the knees, lower back, hands, and hips. Being obese is one of the risk factors of osteoarthritis, among other factors. The excess weight exerts so much pressure on the cartilage and joints, causing them to wear and tear away. Additionally, excess weight often stimulates the release of certain substances that trigger inflammation of the joints and hence, increasing the risk of osteoarthritis.

Fatty Liver Disease

This is also referred to as non-alcoholic steatohepatitis (NASH). It often occurs when the body fats accumulate in the liver, causing injury. It also leads to severe damage of the liver, cirrhosis, and eventually, liver failure.

The thing with this condition is that it produces mild or no symptoms at all. The actual mechanism in which this disease is caused remains unknown. However, the diseases affect obese people as well as those who have diabetes. It is known to affect children and middle-aged adults.

Kidney disease

Kidneys are organs that are bean shaped and are important in filtering blood, getting rid of excess water and waste products in the form of urine. It is also the role of the kidneys to control blood pressure so that the body remains healthy.

Having a kidney disease simply means that the kidneys are damaged in such a way that they cannot filter blood the way they should. It is this can of damage that contributes to the build-up of excess waste in the body. Obesity is known to increase the risk of developing kidney disease. Recent research studies indicate that even in the absence of other risk factors, obesity itself promotes chronic kidney disease and speeds up its progression.

Pregnancy problems

If you are obese or overweight, you may have an increased risk of experiencing various health problems during pregnancy, is you are a mother. This affects both the baby and the mother. This is mainly because, according to research, obese pregnant women are at a higher risk of developing gestational diabetes, preeclampsia, and ultimately requiring a C-section which may cause them to take a long period to recover fully from the operation.

Additionally, babies of women who are obese or overweight have an increased risk of being born preterm or ending up as stillbirths. In other cases, they may even end up having neural tube defects.

One thing that is important to note here is that overweight or obese pregnant women are highly likely to have insulin resistance, high blood pressure, and high sugar levels in the blood. Additionally, obesity increases the time spent performing surgery and hence, increased blood loss. This also has an impact on the baby in the long-term such that they are likely to gain too much weight. Therefore, if you are pregnant, it is advisable that you seek advice from your healthcare provider concerning how much weight gain is right for you during your pregnancy.

Chapter 4 Macronutrients and Micronutrients

Overall, nutrients are divided into two categories: macronutrients and micronutrients. Macronutrients refer to the nutrients that the body needs in large quantities. They are crucial in proving the body with calories or energy; some of the macronutrients include proteins, carbohydrates, and fats. Micronutrients are typically required by the body in smaller amounts; some of the micronutrients include vitamins, minerals, and water. Having established the link between obesity and nutrition choices, it is essential to explore the relationship between the main nutritional categories with obesity. The focus here is to further break down the nutrition-obesity correlation into the finer compositions of dietary choices, with the aim of establishing the contributory aspects of either macro- or micro-nutrients intakes.

Macronutrients

Carbohydrates play a crucial role in the body. Firstly, they fuel the body during high-intensity exercises. Secondly, they are crucial because they help the body to spare body proteins, which is essential in preserving muscle mass during exertions. Thirdly, carbohydrates are the fuel that powers the Central Nervous System (the brain). However, the intake of carbohydrates should be capped at a certain level, consistent with the subject's lifestyle (physical activity). For example, sedentary individuals should take a recommended 40-50 percent of the total calorie daily intake. Individuals that exercise regularly can take up to 60 percent of another total daily calorie intake from carbohydrates. For athletes involved in heavy training, 70 percent of their total daily calorie intake should be from carbs. Some of the primary sources of carbohydrates include grains, dairy products, and fruits.

The intake of carbohydrates is essential in the perspective of obesity because of what the body does to the excess calorie intake. Once the body uses up the required carbohydrates to power the processes and energy-exerting activities, the rest is transformed into sugars and stored in the body. The storage of carbohydrates in the body takes the form of fat tissues, which translates into weight. Therefore, the intake of carbs without a commensurate physical activity or exertion is likely to lead to a surge in an individual's weight.

This highlights the importance of both checking one's intake of carbohydrates and balancing it out with physical activity. At the same time, this underscores the importance of carbohydrate intake, ranging from the functioning of one's brain to the integrity of their body proteins, which are essential in the structure and functioning of the body system as well. However, it is important to highlight the increased correlation between increased carbohydrate and sugars (sugary foods and fizzy drinks) intake and a surge in body weight (obesity). For example, in the US, the statistics regarding obesity, especially among children, has shown an upward trajectory because of the increase in sedentary lifestyles coupled with a surge in the intake of carbohydrates and sugars in the form of fast foods and fizzy drinks.

Proteins play a pivotal role in the human health; they are important in the integrity and structure of boy tissues because they form part of muscles, skin, organ tissues, nails, ligaments, tendons, blood plasma, and hair. Proteins also form part of the cell plasma membranes. They are also involved in the transport, metabolic, and hormone systems. They fundamentally are involved in the regulatory system of metabolism because they make up the enzymes that play this role. Proteins also help in establishing the acid/base balance in the body to maintain a neutral environment for the normal functioning of the human body. The recommended intake of proteins daily is illustrated in the table below:

Lifestyle	Recommended Daily Allowance
Sedentary individuals	Up to 0.36 grams of protein for every pound of body weight
Individuals active recreationally	Between 0.45 and 0.68 grams of protein for every pound of body weight
Competitive athletes	Between 0.54 and 0.82 grams of protein for every pound of body weight
Teenage Athletes	Between 0.82 and 0.91 grams of protein for every pound of body weight
Bodybuilders	Between 0.64 and 0.91 grams of protein for every pound of body weight
Individuals seeking to restrict calories	Between 0.36 and 0.91 grams of protein for every pound of body weight
Optimal utilizable proteins	0.91 grams of protein for every pound of body weight

Some of the sources of proteins from the human diet include meat, some vegetables, animal sources, whole grains such as oats and brown rice, lentils, legumes (beans), soy products (tofu), and seeds.

The role of proteins in the human body is important as underscored above. However, the relationship between the intake of proteins or lack thereof and obesity has not been clearly established in the literature and the field of nutrition and diet. However, the impact of protein intake is mainly influenced by the balance of the diet the subject individual is taking. For example, when taken alongside carbohydrates, proteins have been shown to reduce the gaining of body fat and thus weight. However, excessive intake of proteins can also lead to a surge in body weight as well.

Typically, the common understanding of proteins is that excess intake will not affect body weight because the surplus proteins are excreted, as opposed to what happens to the carbohydrates, which are stored in the body in the form of body fat. However, only excess amino acids are excreted, the rest of the proteins can be stored in the body, and their interaction with the rest of the body nutrients can lead to a surge in body weight as well.

Fats are used in the body as the energy reserve, protecting vital body organs, insulation, and in the transport of fat-soluble vitamins. This highlights the crucial role of fats in the human body, and thus why their intake is essential. Dieticians and nutritionists recommend that beaten 20 and 35 percent of an individual's daily calorie intake should come from fat, but less than 10 percent of the total calorie intake should come from saturated fat from dairy products, full fat, coconut, butter, cream, and cheese.

Fatty foods have been shown to contribute significantly towards the surge in body weight. In many cases, a fat-reduced diet leads to an average loss of weight of between 3 and 4 kilograms compared to the typical-fat diets. A 10 percent reduction of dietary fat can lead to a weight loss of between 4 and 5 kilograms. This highlights a strong correlation between the amount of dietary fat intake and obesity. In this regard, people taking excessive dietary fat are likely to gain weight and thus become obese compared to people with reduced dietary fat intakes.

Micronutrients

Micronutrients, such as vitamins and minerals, play a crucial role in the functioning of the body systems and human health as a whole. Regarding obesity, the most important aspect affected by micronutrients is the metabolism process. In many cases, metabolism has a direct impact on the body's consumption of energy and its ability to store down excess energy in the form of body fat. At the same time, metabolism determines the utilization of body fat – which directly affects the loss of weight. Therefore, this underscores the importance of micronutrients in affects human nutrition as well as the gaining or losing body weight.

For example, vitamin D deficiency has been reported among obese individuals and in diabetics. Dieticians and nutritionists have asserted that there is an essential health benefit in vitamin D supplementation, which helps the overall body metabolic system to establish a balanced energy utilization and storage balance. Among diabetics, the deficiency of Chromium, an essential trace metal required in the signaling of the insulin cascade, leads to increased predisposition to weight gain and diabetes as well. Moreover, a biotin deficiency, a water-soluble cofactor essential in the enzymatic breakdown of fatty acids, affects the metabolism of proteins, which disrupts the body's weight gain and loss balance as well.

The highlight here is that micronutrients play a crucial role in the regulatory process of the body's metabolism as a whole, which in turn influences the body's ability to utilize energy and store excess energy in the form of body fat and thus lead to weight gain. Therefore, the intake of micronutrients is especially important in maintaining a low weight or in the process of losing weight as well. Individuals with a reduced intake of micronutrients face an increased likelihood of gaining weight and vice versa.

Chapter 5 Portion control

According to the National Institute of Health, food portions in the US have increased by 50 percent over the last two decades. The institute highlights this alarming statistic as the baseline for the surge in obesity rates among both children and adults. In this regard, the rise in the size of meals, and the ubiquitous nature of the super-sized meals across American means that more and more people have a hard time determining and recognizing proper portions as well as serving sizes. This underscores the importance of controlling portions; whether you want to lose a few pounds or just maintain a healthy weight, it is as important to eat proper portions as it is to eat the right foods and balance the diet. In this regard, a portion is the total amount of food that an individual eats in one sitting. Therefore, the doubling of the portion sizes over the last 20 years means that more and more Americans are eating more food that they require for their dietary needs. This means that excess intake of food leads to a surge in the amount of excel nutrients the body stores in the form of body fat. As a result, this has a direct bearing on the rise in the number of people facing obesity among adults as well as children.

Portion control involves several approaches and methods employed to control the amount of food an individual takes within one setting. For example, measuring food is important because it helps a person to see the amount they eat. It also controls the portions one eats, which helps reduce instances of overeating.

Using smaller dishware is also another tactic that helps in providing an individual a measure of control how much food they eat, while also adjusting the portion downwards. A smaller plate makes the food seem larger, which helps cultivate the feeling of satiety, without necessary overeating – it is a small and typically effective trick to the stomach. Serving food separately also helps in reducing the risk of taking too much food from a large plate, which will keep the portion taken under control. Packaging food into single and measured portions helps one to regulate the amount of food they eat from the fridge; it also reminds one that a single package is sufficient, which reduces the temptation of overeating. Adding more vegetables, for example, eating a salad before a meal will reduce the amount of food one eventually eats. It also helps one to control their portions. At the same time, including veggies in sandwiches helps in making one feel full without necessarily eating more calories.

These tactics highlight that the target of portion control is reducing the amount of food one eats, which in turn controls the number of nutrients (carbohydrates, proteins, fats, vitamins, and minerals) that one ends up in-taking into their body. These nutrients have a demonstrable influence on the issue of weight and health of a person. Therefore, balancing the amount of intake (size of the portion) with physical activity or lifestyle is essential in maintaining a healthy weight. Otherwise, this either leads to excessive weight gain (obesity) or loss, both of which pose considerable health risks to the affected individual.

The doubling of portion sizes in recent years means that a significant chunk of people do not consider the amount of food they take in one sitting. This means that most of them end up eating beyond the amount their body requires in maintaining their health and performance. Without developing or sustaining the culture of checking and ascertaining the portion control culture, this has affected the children as well, with their intake of carbohydrates, fats, and proteins. In this regard, most of them do not understand or know how to check for feelings of satiety. As a result, they tend to go over the limit with the amounts they eat, which predisposes them to gain weight and thus, obesity. This is especially the case with the increase depositions of carbohydrates and fats, intakes that have been established to have a strong correlation with gaining weight and obesity. This highlights the importance of portion control – some of the crucial aspects of diet and health that necessitate portion control are discussed below:

Reducing Binge Eating

Binge eating means an excessive intake of food and nutrients into the body. However, portion control plays a crucial role in controlling the amount of food an individual takes in one setting, which helps in making the stomach smaller. The target here is creating an overarching habit of eating a specific amount of food (portion) in one setting, which is essential in controlling or reducing food craving. It helps the individual to connect acutely with their senses of satiety, which is crucial in stopping eating food once the required minimum for the health and performance of the body is met. In the process, this approach helps in eliminating the process of binge eating, establishing more control on the amount of food one needs, and also developing sharp senses of satiety, which will help in reducing the amount of food intake beyond the required nutritive value by the body.

Glucose Level Balance

The favored metabolic pathway of the body typically involves the breakdown of consumed food into glucose – the entry substrate into the metabolic pathways. In this regard, the increased intake of food, in the form of super-sized portions, leads to a constant increase in body glucose – the more one eats, the more glucose gets into the body. Therefore, overeating causes a jumping of the level of glucose, and thus eventually leads to problems such as hypo-/hyperglycaemia and diabetes.

Portion control allows one to establish a stable amount of food, a balanced diet that will sustain their daily lives and their body nutritional requirements. This way, they can maintain any excessive intake of food, which will help keep the body glucose at sable and healthy levels as well.

Bolstering Satiety

Contrary to the widespread perceptions in society, eating less makes an individual feel full faster. This is typical because the stomach shrinks to adjust to the amount of food that the individual takes. Therefore, this establishes a direct link between satiety and portion control. In this case, portion control sets a stable amount of food that a person takes. In response, the stomach shrinks to meet this level, which makes the established portion as the sufficient amount for satiety. Moreover, satiety comes fast soon after one starts eating, which helps in reducing the amount of food one takes overall, which is crucial in preventing overeating, and this keeping calorie intake to within the norm.

Weight Loss or Maintaining a Healthy Weight

This aspect establishes the importance of portion control in regulating, managing, or addressing obesity, which is the highlight of this book. As found in the macronutrient and micronutrient section above, there is a close correlation between the amount of food one takes and their predisposition to gaining weight and developing obesity. As a result, this highlights the importance of portion control as a fundamental approach to preventing weight gain, losing weight, or maintaining a healthy weight.

In losing weight, making the eating portions smaller is a major priority. In many cases, obesity is occasioned by the excessive intake of foods and nutrients into the body that the body does not necessarily need. This is especially the case among the people with sedentary lifestyles and reduced exertions. Most of the carbohydrates, proteins, and fats they eat are not used up because they experience little physical activities. As a result, the eating of large portions means that most of the nutrients are stored in the body, which increases their chances of gaining weight and progressing to obesity if no action is taken.

Portion control allows the individual to be in control of their food intake, instead of being dictated to by their habits and cravings. As a result, the individual with portion control will not feel hungry and crave junk food. Instead, they have an increased measure of control over what, where, and when they eat. It also allows the individual to condition the body to eat a healthy diet which provides sufficient protein, fats, and carbohydrates.

Chapter 6 Obesity Myths

In recent years, the surge in obesity among adults and children, and the accompanying health effects and cost have led to a rise in attention and focus on this disorder from the government, private sector, and the general public. However, increased scrutiny has also led to a steady supply of myths, misconceptions, and misunderstandings. Some of the myths regarding obesity are discussed below.

Myth 1- Genes are to Blame for Obesity

According to the Washington Post, as obesity rates have increased markedly in the US, researchers have focused on determining a link between the genetic makeup of obese people and their ability or predisposition to gaining weight and eventually developing obesity. However, this disproportional focus on genetics is not consistent with the obesity trend – between the year 1980 and 2000, the number of people in America that are obese has increased by 50 percent. This shift is too quick to be driven by genetic predisposition among obese people and their families.

Therefore, people do not eat more than they need because they are genetically predisposed to eating that way; instead, people overeat because they can. One dollar is putting more calories on the table than ever before, which means that people have access to more food portions at home, fast food outlets, and restaurants. Additionally, more people are dining away from their homes than ever. In 1966, the average family's expenses on its food budget away from home were pegged at 31 percent. This surged to 49 percent in 2011. Therefore, the nutritional correlation to obesity is more plausible compared to genetic assertions.

The food industry's business model has focused on developing thousands of food products in the market with massive amounts of calories for every bite. They have also devised effective marketing strategic approaches that have convinced an increasing number of people to purchase and consume these foods, typically more than their baseline nutritional requirements. This further underscores the link between nutrition and obesity as opposed to the relationship between genetics and predisposition to obesity.

Myth 2 - Lack of Self-Control is Responsible for Obesity

A study conducted by Utrecht University has proven that "*dieting, in most circumstances, is not a feasible strategy in managing weight.*" In this regard, the myth is that people with self-control can control the amount of food they eat, which will translate to losing weight or maintaining a steady, healthy weight. However, this study indicates that such control does not typically lead to loss of weight. This myth does not establish the role played by the overall environment, mental state, and other influences affect what people eat and how much they eat as well.

The overall reality is that the modern world is filled with calorie-styled temptations that we can be led to consuming too much in ways that we do not understand. The food industry companies have worked with psychologists to come up with targeted marketing approaches, which increase people's consumption of calorie-filled foods; as a result, obesity is driven by the overarching culture in the community as opposed to pegging it on the self-control of individuals.

Additionally, this myth is design to be discriminatory towards people with obesity, as opposed to recognizing the underlying and societal challenge surrounding eating habits, the food industry, and the correlations they have towards the societal problem with weight gain and obesity among adults and children.

Myth 3 - The Obesity Epidemic is driven by a Lack of Access to Fresh Vegetables and Fruits

The Healthy Food Financing Initiative, developed under the Obama administration in the US, was designed to help low-income communities to gain access to healthy fresh food. According to the US Department of Agriculture, less than 5 percent of the people in America live in these "food deserts," while about 65 percent of the US population is overweight or obese. However, the zeroing in on fresh vegetables and fruits as the underlying cause of obesity does not ring true because a massive number of Americans have the choice between fresh fruits and vegetables on the one hand and the other the convenient and tasty fast/junk foods dominating the market and local outlets.

Obesity usually results from overeating junk food and eating bigger portions than is required for the standard dietary requirements.

People might head to the grocery section with good intentions of purchasing healthy foods. However, when confronted by candy at the cash register, they end up purchasing the 'unhealthy' food, not because they do not have access to fresh fruits and vegetables, but because of the prevailing mentality, attitudinal, and behavioral inclinations regarding purchase and eating habits.

Most of the food retailers have created a sharpened over time impulse-marketing strategies to significantly influence purchase behavior and thus eating habits. This is more of a contributor towards obesity across the population, not just for the people that cannot access fresh vegetables and fruits, but also among those that can access them but choose to purchase junk fast foods. Therefore, although Obama's Healthy Food Financing Initiative was effective in expanding the nutritional portfolio of many of these disadvantaged communities; it missed the mark on obesity, and thus helped entrench this myth in the society.

Myth 4 - It is not overeating that Causes Obesity, but it is leading a too Sedentary Lifestyle

In 2013, the then First lady Michele Obama launched a campaign called "Let's Move," which was based on the idea that if kids exercised more, the US could make inroads in addressing the issue of childhood obesity. However, according to the Centres for Disease Control and Prevention, the trends between the 1980s and 1990s, when the obesity rates soared, were not accompanied by a decline in physical activity. Although work-related physical activities saw a considerable drop, leisure-related physical activities increased markedly. According to the National Health and Nutrition Examination, on average, people take in around 500 more calories every day now in 2019 as compared to what they consumed in the late 1970s before obesity rates surged. This underscores compelling correlation between surges in the intake of calories for the increasing obesity cases as opposed to the sedentary lifestyle.

Therefore, the "Let's Move" campaign, although well intentioned, helps to establish the myth that the increasing obesity levels in the US among children and adults is as a result of a decline in physical activity. Instead, the truth here is that the surge of obesity levels in the US over the last two decades has had more to do with the choices in nutrition as opposed to physical activity. This is especially because there has not been any demonstrable net reduction of physical activity, even despite the lifestyle changes in recent years.

Myth 5 – Better Education Regarding Diet and Nutrition can help in Conquering Obesity

A study carried out on physician's health conducted by the American Family Physician in 2007 reveals that 44 percent of male doctors in the US are overweight. A survey conducted by the University of Maryland's School of Nursing revealed that 55 percent of all the surveyed nurses were overweight or obese. The question here is – if people providing healthcare services cannot control their weight, why would a focus on education of nutrition and diet lead to any difference for others in the community?

Inundating the people with more information about extra-large portions, sophisticated marketing messaging, and food, the ability of such people to limit their consumption of food and eating habits is considerably restricted. This is underscored by the general lack of restrictions on the eating habits among people in America, as compared to the significant restrictions placed on drinking alcohol in the country including age limits at 21 years and that alcohol cannot be sold through vending machines.

Comparatively, in the 19th century, an era where control on the quality and consumption of drinking water was not advanced, the population was widely affected by infectious diseases, which became major causes of death. Once the standards were established, and the sector regulated strictly, the deaths plummeted, and the safety of the population was bolstered. Therefore, there is a need for expanded regulation regarding eating habits in the country, with the aim of establishing a healthy eating habit in the nation, and thus preventing many Americans from facing the consequences of obesity and predisposition to the accompanying disorders. Although education can help tackle the issue of obesity, establish that knowledge regarding diet and nutrition is a panacea in reducing and eliminating obesity is not supported by fact, and thus a myth.

Myth 6 – Carbohydrates are Bad, Get Rid of them from the Diet

The myth here is that for one to become healthier, lose weight, or maintain a healthy weight, they have to get rid of all the carbohydrates from their diets. However, this is not consistent with the fact, which highlights the importance of carbohydrates to the functioning of the body. Taken as part of a healthy and balanced diet, carbohydrates are not all bad. Moreover, most of the healthy foods such as vegetables and fruits are rich in carbohydrates. Some of the dangers of carbs are underscored by the processed and added sugars in some carb types such as white bread, which are more damaging and should be avoided.

Therefore, placing a blanket declaration on all carbs that "they are unhealthy" is not representative of fact, and is inconsistent with nutritionists and dieticians' recommendations regarding a balanced diet. The overall concept here is that there is a need for individuals to control the amount of food (portions) they eat relative to their physical activity. Obesity is brought about by a series of several factors and not a single issue. This means that the approaches to address these issues should be multi-faceted as well.

Chapter 7 Role of Diet

One of the main goals of having a proper diet is to ensure that you do not put on more weight. This means that you have to come up with realistic weight-loss goals you can work hard to attain. It is important that you realize that the ideal weight has to have a corresponding BMI of between 20 and 25. In spite of the fact that this may seem like something easy to achieve on paper, practically, it is something that so many people find to be challenging. Your first objective should be to lose at least 15% of your current weight as opposed to targeting over 20% of your weight. Just remember that losing weight is accompanied by so many health benefits for any person that is obese.

The easiest and most effective means to weight loss is through consumption of fewer calories. To lose a pound, you need to burn at least 3,500 calories. For an adult, the daily caloric intake is 1200-2800 calories/day, taking into consideration the level of activity and the body size to satisfy the energy needs of the body.

In other words, if you lose a pound each week, it is reasonable and very safe rather than overworking to lose too much weight at once. What is interesting is that the higher your starting weight, the faster you can achieve weight loss. The main reason for this is that for every kilogram of body weight, you need at least 22 calories to maintain that weight. Therefore, if you are 100 kilograms, you will need at least 2200 calories daily to maintain that body weight. However, you have to notice that several other factors determine the caloric expenditure, such as age. In other words, as one grows older, the metabolic rate slows down, making it harder to shed some weight.

Here are some of the general guidelines you can follow to maintain healthy body weight;

For one to maintain a safe and healthy body weight in the long-term, it is critical that they consume a diet that contains a balanced and nutritious diet. This ensures that the body has an adequate supply of both macros- and micronutrients and hence preventing malnutrition diseases.

The other trick is to ensure that your diet is composed largely of nutritious foods low in energy density. This is mainly because low-energy dense foods have few amounts of calories per unit weight. For instance, vegetables, lean meat, beans, fruits, fish, and grains are some of the foods that are said to be low energy dense. In other words, you can take a large amount of celery and beans without necessarily consuming too many calories.

On the other hand, it is also important that you cut down on energy-dense foods, mainly because of their high fat and simple sugar content. In other words, when you consume these foods, you take in lots of calories in a small portion of food. According to the U.S. government, it is recommended that for any to be considered healthy, it has to have less than 30% fat content mainly because fats contain at least two times as much calories per unit weight compared to proteins and carbs.

For instance, egg yolk, sweets, butter, high-fat salad dressing, red meat, fried foods, and pastries, among others are some of the high energy dense foods. Therefore, it is important that you reduce your intake of foods loaded with calories and replace them with nutritious low-calorie foods.

You have to understand that approximately 55% of calories in a diet should be complex carbs. Therefore, eat as many complex carbs as you can. You can find this in brown rice, vegetables, fruits, and whole-grain bread. In other words, try as much as possible to stay away from simple carbs like doughnuts, muffins, and cakes, among others. Also, cut down on sugary drinks because they are loaded with simple sugars. It is these simple sugars that cause the pancreas to release excessive amounts of insulin, hence promoting the growth of fat tissues.

Additionally, before you can start shopping and filling your trolley or shopping cart with food products, ensure that you read the labels to estimate how much calories there are in a serving size. Finally, ensure that you consult your dietician, nutritionist, or healthcare professional to determine how much calories you should consume in a diet daily

Role of medication in the treatment of obesity

It is important to note that obesity medication should be used by people with a BMI of above 30. However, it is important that you also seek medical advice before you can take any weight loss medications. These medications should be used as part of a diet modification or a workout program.

If the medication is successful, then you expect to lose at least 6 pounds in the first month and eventually lose a total weight of between 10 and 15 %. If you discontinue the medication, weight gain is likely to occur, hence the need to keep taking them as long as you need to lose weight.

One thing that is also important to note is that the first class of medications plays a critical role in weight control, and often are known to induce certain symptoms that trigger the sympathetic nervous system. In other words, they induce stress and anxiety. As a result of this, the patient may start having side effects of hypertension. Some of these class of medications include phentermine and sibutramine, among others.

The other thing is that these first-class medications often cause a reduction in appetite by creating a strong sensation of satiety. It is the role of certain neurotransmitters to regulate both hunger and satiety. Some of these neurotransmitters include; serotonin, dopamine, and norepinephrine. Therefore, the main role of medications against obesity is to ensure that they suppress appetite by simply stimulating the increase of these neurotransmitters located on the synapse (junction between the nerve endings in the brain).

Phentermine

This is also referred to as Fatin or Adipex P. Its main role is to suppress one's appetite by stimulating an increased in the release of norepinephrine. It is important in treating obesity in the short-term. Its common side effects include irritability, headaches, insomnia, and anxiety.

On the other hand, Fenfluramine and dexfenfluramine play a critical role in increasing the levels of serotonin in the body and hence, suppressing appetite. However, the problem is that these two drugs were withdrawn because they were shown to cause pulmonary hypertension, a serious disease of the arteries located in the lungs.

Since, some people have suggested that a combination of phentermine with fluoxetine, something referred to as Phen/pro. The problem with this is that there are no clinical trials that demonstrate their safety and effectiveness when used in combination. Therefore, this is not accepted for use in the treatment of obesity.

Orlistat

This is referred to as Xenical or all. It falls in the second category of drugs that work by altering the fat metabolism in the body. It is also the only drug that is currently being used and has been approved by the U.S. FDA. They are simply known as lipase inhibitors or fat blockers.

What is interesting is that the facts from foods can only be absorbed into the bloodstream once they have been digested by a group of enzymes referred to as lipases, located in the intestines. Therefore, by inhibiting the action of these enzymes, this drug prevents the intestines from absorbing fats by about 30%.

The good thing with this drug is the fact that they do not affect the chemistry of the brain. In theory, they are also known to have no systemic side effects mainly because their location of action is the gut lumen, and very little of this drug is absorbed into the blood system. Once it was approved by the FDA, this drug was branded alli and sold over the counter for the treatment of obesity since February 2007.

Additionally, this drug is recommended for use by people who are 18 years and above and can be used in combination with an exercise and diet program. Therefore, if you are not of age, and are not overweight (BMI of 27 and above), then there is no way you should be allowed to take orlistat.

This drug is to be taken three times a day with a fat-containing food. You can take it during meals or an hour after meals. If you miss a meal, or the meal you are taking is very low in fat content, then there is no need for you to take the medication.

Some of the most common side effects of this drug include changes in the habits of the bowel. In other words, the patient often experiences gas, urgent desire to have a bowel movement, frequency in bowel movement, as well as the inability to control the movement of the bowel. With women, there are cases or irregular menstrual flow, and this is evident during the first few weeks of starting the medication. In other people, these side effects persist for as long as they continue to take the medication.

It is also important to note that if you have a thyroid condition or are diabetic, have received an organ transplant or are under medication that affects blood clotting; it is highly recommended that you check with your doctor/physician before you can start on the orlistat medication, to avoid any possible drug interactions. In other cases, patients develop a deficiency of fat-soluble vitamins like A, D, E, and K. In such a situation, it is important that these patients are started in vitamin supplements.

Role of weight loss surgery in the treatment of obesity

According to the NIH, certain guidelines have been set in place for weight-loss surgery for patients with obesity. One study compared the rate at which hypertension and diabetes occurred in two groups each having obese patients. One of the groups underwent weight loss surgery while the other did not. Each of the groups has a similar starting. After two years, what was interesting was that the occurrence of diabetes and hypertension was reduced in patients who had had weight loss surgery. If you are obese and have a surgical procedure performed on your upper GIT, these procedures are collectively referred to as bariatric surgery.

The very first surgeries to be performed included the jejunocolic and jejunoileal bypass. In such a case, the small bowel is simply diverted to the large one, such that it bypasses a large surface area of food absorption. However, some problems arose with these procedures and their use was discontinued.

Currently, some of the weight loss surgical procedures being used include making the stomach area quite small or entirely bypassing the stomach. There two procedures actively being used;

- Restrictive surgeries that specifically limits the size of the stomach while also slowing down the rate of digestion.
- Malabsorptive surgeries that play a significant role in restricting the stomach. It also bypasses or otherwise gets rid of some part of the digestive system to lower absorption of foods and hence low amounts of calories.

One of the most common malabsorptive surgery is referred to as the Roux-en-Y gastric bypass. Here, the stomach is slightly stapled so that it creates something like a pouch. In this case, part of the intestine is attached to the pouch formed to lower the rate of food absorption.

That said, surgical treatments of obesity are constantly evolving and are often performed using the laparoscopic methods. In other words, they use tiny incisions along with a camera in performing the actual surgery. In spite of the fact that these surgical procedures are slowly becoming routine, the rate of mortality for them is still at 2% with a high possibility of one developing complications.

Some of the risks associated with these surgical procedures include the common complications brought by infections, developing clots in the lungs as well as lower extremities of the body and possibility of an increased anesthesia risk. Some of the long-term risks include iron deficiency anemia and insufficient iron absorption. Patients have also been reported to have Vitamin B12 deficiency and damage to the nerves (neuropathies). It is important to bear in mind that when you lose weight rapidly, the chances are that you might develop gallstones. It is advisable that these bariatric surgical procedures are performed at an institution with a weight-loss program that has employed licenced dieticians to ensure proper follow-up of patients.

Are meal substitutes, artificial sweeteners, and over-the-counter (OTC) products effective in treating obesity?

This is one of the questions that so many people with obesity ask. Well, the truth is;

Meal substitutes

When these are used as regular meals or substitutes, they can be very convenient in lowering the caloric-intake as part of the whole low-calorie diet plan. One of the common meals substitutes available in powder form is the Slim-Fast. The other one available in both liquid form and bars is referred to as Ensure.

It is important that when you choose to take meal substitutes, they offer proteins, low levels of fats, and low amounts of calories. To find more details about the number of calories in every serving as well as the proportion of macronutrients, it is critical that you check the label. If the amount is already predetermined, then it is much easier to keep track of your daily intake. Just like any other dramatic change in your diet, it is advisable that you consult a professional healthcare provider before you can incorporate these changes into your lifestyle so that you are aware of any negative effects that might come with its use.

Artificial Sweeteners

Some of the common examples of artificial sweeteners include Saccharins and Aspartame. They simply serve as substitutes of sugars with very low levels or no calorie content. In other cases, people use them as a substitute for normal table sugar. When you use Saccharin in place of a teaspoon of sugar, you are essentially getting rid of the amount 33 calories from your diet.

If you have phenylketonuria, it is advisable that you avoid using Aspartame as it contains Phenylalanine. Other sugar alternatives you can choose to use include sorbitol and xylitol. However, they provide a higher caloric content compared to both Aspartame and Saccharin. Note that excessive use of sorbitol may contribute to the occurrence of diarrhea.

Over-the-counter weight-loss products

Even though there have been so many claims by manufacturers, you have to understand that using OTC weight-loss products alone will not help you lose weight. What is even more misleading is that certain herbal weight-loss products are referred to as fat burners and do not help lose weight safely and healthily. This is mainly because these products are loaded with ma huang, Hoodia gordonia, white willow, and kola nut. All these components are stimulants that increase the rate of metabolism and helps the body burn fats.

Nevertheless, there are no scientific findings that serve as evidence for their effectiveness in weight loss. Additionally, the substance ma huang has been linked to having very serious side effects like seizures, heart attack, and ultimately, death. Chromium, a very popular product in these weight loss products has not been shown to have effects on weight loss.

On the other hand, there are so many weight loss teas that contain strong botanical laxatives and diuretics that have been shown to contribute to water loss from the body and diarrhea. It is these effects that contribute to the depletion of potassium and sodium electrolytes in the body and hence leading to dehydration. In spite of the fact that one will lose weight, the loss is not healthy but rather causes a reduction in the number of fluids in the body, and this is just a temporary undertaking.

Another product that has been commonly used for weight loss is guar gum preparation. It is thought that this preparation works by stimulating feelings of satiety early in the meal. This is not something that has been proven scientifically. However, it is known to cause gas, abdominal cramps, and diarrhea.

All the OTC products we have discussed here are not considered to be drugs and hence, have not to be approved by the FDA. Because of this, there is a limited amount of information on the safety and effectiveness associated with its usage. Therefore, before you can decide to use these OTC products, it is important that you discuss your intentions with a healthcare professional.

Chapter 8 Healthy Eating Plan

Healthy eating is not something easy. It requires so much commitment to a healthy diet, and you will thank yourself later for making a smart decision. Why is that? Well, the truth is, healthy eating will not only make you lose some pounds and make you look and feel better, but it will also save you lots of money that you would have otherwise spent on future health costs.

Yes, you want to start eating healthy so that you can lose weight and lower your risk of developing serious diseases, but do you know what exactly it means to eat healthily? Following a healthy diet plan is about incorporating plenty of vegetables, fruits, whole grains, and other diets into your meal plan. Healthy eating is also about getting rid of foods that are loaded with lots of calories per serving, sugars, and saturated fats.

So, what is it that will help get you motivated to eat healthily and get back your body weight to normal? Here are some of the reasons;

Weight regulation

The main reason why you are reading this book is to help you gain a deeper understanding of obesity, among other reasons. However, in spite the fact that we know the importance of losing weight and maintaining healthy normal body weight, it is still critical that it is mentioned as one of the reasons to adopt a healthy eating plan.

You have to remember that, more than half of the American population is either overweight or obese, and it is the major contributing factor to serious diseases that ultimately lead to death. It is through a healthy diet that you can lose weight, lower your blood pressure, improve your cholesterol levels, and reduce the risk of developing type 2 diabetes.

It takes simple health choices to attain healthy body weight. These simple choices include giving up sodas for water, choosing vegetables over chips, among others. In addition to helping you lose weight, you will save lots of money. According to a survey conducted by the Journal of Health Economics between 2000 and 2005, an average obese person is said to spend at least $2,750 more on health care annually compared to someone with normal body weight.

Increase productivity

Just like a machine, the body and the brain need quality fuel for them to run efficiently. As far as your job and profession are concerned, working efficiently will help boost your productivity and earn you much more money. In other words, you will be on the first line for a raise or a promotion.

One study conducted in 2012 and published in the Journal of Population Health Management reported that consuming a diet that in unhealthy places one at 66% risk of losing productivity. Another study published in the Journal of Occupational and Environmental Medicine reported that consuming an unhealthy diet represents the highest risk of reduced productivity out of 19 other risk factors.

Save money on life insurance

One thing that people fail to understand is that health insurance premiums cannot in any way be based on health factors, and is the reason why each one of us is required to have a health insurance cover. However, of importance is the fact age and health condition on an individual play a key role in their life insurance rates.

Therefore, if you are trying to get the best life insurance, there is a high chance that your insurer will be interested in looking at your medical records, and in most cases even ask for a life insurance medical examination. If you are obese, the chances are that you will spend even more than double the cost of life insurance. It is advisable you decide to switch to a healthier diet and maintain a healthy body weight before you can apply for life insurance, hence lowering the cost of your policy significantly.

Enhance mood

Did you know that what you eat has a great impact on the parts of your brain responsible for mood regulation? Even though no one food has been proven as an antidepressant, proper nutrition is important in ensuring that the blood sugar level is stable so that you can generally feel better on most days. Studies have shown that foods rich in vitamins and minerals such as vegetables, whole grains and fruits lowers the risk of developing depression just like foods loaded with omega-3 fatty acids, e.g., salmon, nuts and other fatty fishes.

The truth is, for you to have true happiness, it is not just about the absence of depression. It involves your entire well-being. It is about your ability to pay attention to important things after changing your diet plan to a healthy pattern of eating.

When you eat healthily, you are in effect lowering the risk of stress. This is because, if your body is in a chronic state of stress, there is a high likelihood that proteins will be broken down in readiness for fight and flight. However, there are certain foods that can moderate the stress hormone called cortisol.

Certain studies have shown that consuming foods rich in omega-3 fatty acids as well as magnesium are important in lowering the levels of cortisol. On the other hand, consuming foods rich in proteins like fish and dairy products play a role in replenishing protein stores and keeping the levels of cortisol low.

Be healthier

Well, it is common for us to see someone who is thin and quickly think that they are healthy. On the other hand, we look at someone big and judge that they are obese when it may be just that they are muscular, but their body fat levels are normal. That said, eating healthy can improve one's health even for people who are thin and still take lots of junk foods (anything that has a high caloric content and low micronutrients) like greasy foods and sodas.

You have to remember that, when you miss out on vitamins and minerals the body requires, you place yourself at risk of early death. According to a study conducted in 2014, it is evident that eating at least five servings of fruit and vegetables each day lowers the risk of early deaths among other health-related problems.

Foods: The Good and Bad

Well, it is true that no food is a magic bullet for weight loss. However, certain foods go a long way in helping one achieve their weight loss goals. What you will notice is that most of these foods have some things in common; high fiber content and low energy density. This simply means that you can eat a decent portion without necessarily exaggerating the number of calories consumed. Here are some of the foods that are good for your weight-loss plan;

Avocados

They are rich in monounsaturated fatty acids, potassium, fiber, and phytochemicals. Research shows that people who eat avocados often have a lower BMI, waist circumference, and body weight compared to those who choose to skip it altogether. While this green superfood is loaded with high-calorie content compared to other fruits, it is their fat content and fiber combo that makes it satisfying and helps one slim down. Integrate this to your diet for a burst of flavor and creaminess.

Eggs

They are rich in high-quality proteins, essential nutrients, and fats. The good news about eggs is that the protein it has and the time of day we eat them makes them perfect powerhouses for weight loss.

When you have an egg for breakfast, the protein increases satiety and regulates hunger and appetite hormones.

Beans

Beans are rich in fiber, making it your best friend when you are obese and looking to lose weight. When you eat beans, it keeps you fuller for longer and hence controls hunger pangs. According to research, consuming beans and legumes, in general, is linked to so many health benefits such as lowering the blood pressure, reducing the risk of developing heart disease, lowering the levels of LDL cholesterol in the blood.

Yogurt

They are packed with proteins and probiotics that are good for your gut health. They also help in weight loss. One thing that you have to understand is that your gut health influences your weight. Therefore, when you consume high amounts of fiber and probiotics, your gut microbiome is happy, and this is a good thing for your metabolism.

If you want to eat lots of proteins, choose the Greek Yoghurt, which is also associated with reduced appetite and keeping you fuller for longer. However, it is important that you watch out for added sugars in flavored yogurts, which tends to add extra calories back into your diet. If you want to sweeten, you can use natural fresh fruits, which adds an extra kick of flavor and nutrition.

Salmon

They are rich in good omega-3 fatty acids and high-quality proteins. A diet that is loaded with omega-3 fatty acids plays a key role in increasing one's satiety, especially if you are obese and looking to lose weight. It is recommended that you have at least two servings of salmon every week.

Fruits

One thing that makes fruits a bad rap sometimes is the fact that they contain sugars. However, eating fruits can go a long way in helping you lose weight, especially when you incorporate fruits in your diet plan to replace processed and unhealthy snacks. They are also loaded with lots of fiber that keeps you satisfied for longer. Plus, you get an extra kick of antioxidants that boosts your immune system while also lowering your risk of gaining more weight and becoming overweight or obese.

Almonds

They are loaded with fiber and proteins. When you eat foods that are loaded with fiber and proteins, you will stay fuller for longer, which reduces the temptation of reaching for unhealthy cravings. They are also a good source of Vitamin E and mono- as well as polyunsaturated fatty acids. You can add them to your salads, side dishes or topping up your morning granola and you are good to go.

That said, one thing that you have to note is that eating unhealthy diets does not just mean eating unhealthy meals. It also means having a low amount of nutrients in your diet, hence contributing to obesity. It also means that you are taking in too much energy by eating lots of calories and not burning them.

Some of the foods that contribute to excessive weight gain especially when you do not engage in regular physical activities include;

- Foods and drinks that are loaded with high levels of sugars and calories
- Foods that have low amounts of proteins and fiber
- Foods that are made from refined carbs like white bread

According to research scientists, the most important thing is emphasizing on portion control as we have already discussed in this book. It seems obvious just to say that eating too much will make you gain more weight and become obese or overweight. However, so many people do not take into consideration how much they eat, especially when selecting the foods to eat.

Bear in mind that excessive intake of calories regardless of the source increases the chance of putting on more weight, especially if you are not expending that energy through regular workouts. However, that is not to say that the food composition you eat does not count. It is better if you eat whole grains, vegetables, and fruits rather than fried chicken and potato fries. You have to emphasize on a balanced diet made up of proteins, fiber, and overall, few calories to make a real difference.

Healthy Eating Tips

Trust me, if adopting a healthy diet was something easy, each one of us would have done it, and we would not be talking about here in this manner. Therefore, if you are experiencing a hard time choosing the right food and sticking to a healthy diet plan, take some pressure off yourself. Do not aim for big milestones at the same time. Take small baby steps, and over time, you will appreciate how much they pay off.

In other words, it is important that you set small milestones that you can attain, and eventually, they will all translate to long-term outcomes. Here are some tips that will help you eat healthily and keep that weight off for a very long time;

- Hydrate as much as you can to help lower your cravings will keep you full for longer
- Instead of skipping meals, ensure that you eat at about the same time each day as much as you can
- Ensure that you are physically active as this has been shown to create a mindset of healthy eating too
- Always plan around cravings early enough so that you do not end up eating foods that are not healthy for your body
- We are all human; therefore, forgive yourself when you slip. Beating yourself up for that bowl of ice-cream or bag of potato chips will tend to unravel most of your goals. Pick right up and keep pressing on towards your goals

That said, always bear in mind that healthy eating is a good choice that happens one bit at a time. Start by making a few small changes in the right direction as this will help improve your life little by little until you eventually achieve all of your health goals.

Conclusion

There has been significant research work that has been done towards understanding obesity as well as improving the treatment of this condition. With time, there will be better, safer, and more effective strategies for the treatment of obesity. However, currently, there is no magic pill that cures obesity.

The best and the safest means by which one can overcome obesity and keep that weight off is through a commitment to a lifelong process of regular exercise and proper diet plan. All the medications we have discussed above are supposed to be considered as adjuncts to exercise and diet because the health risk from obesity far much outweighs the effects of the medications.

Additionally, it is important that these medications are prescribed by the doctor who is well informed about your health history as well as the use of medications. It is also important that all other medications and preparations that have not been approved by the FDA be avoided by all means possible.

What you have to understand is that there are five features of a successful weight-loss programs that you should look out for. These features include;

- A safe diet with all the recommended daily allowances (RDA) for vitamins, proteins, and minerals.
- A weight-loss program directed towards a slow but steady weight loss, unless your Physician advises that your health condition might benefit from a rapid weight loss.

- Before starting a weight-loss, the program should evaluate your health condition or ensure that you take your medication regularly, especially if you plan on losing between 15 and 20 pounds.
- Have a plan for weight-loss maintenance after the whole phase of weight-loss is over. Trust me; there is no use of losing a significant amount of weight only to regain it after a short time. In as much as this is the most difficult phases of them all, it is one of the areas that are not implemented consistently in weight-loss programs. Therefore, ensure that the program you choose offers adequate help in changing your dietary habits permanently and improving your physical activity into the long-term. Try as much as you can to engage in exercises throughout the day so that you can burn as many calories as possible.
- Finally, if you are enrolled in a commercial weight-loss program, it should provide you with a detailed statement of the amount to be paid as fee including all other additional costs like purchasing dietary supplements among others.

You have to realize that obesity is not something small; it is a chronic condition. It is unfortunate that too often, people think of obesity as a temporary problem that can just be treated within a few days with a harsh diet. However, if you are going to lose weight and have healthy body weight, then you have to look at this as a lifelong effort. Therefore, ensure that the weight-loss program you choose offers a long-term strategy. Otherwise, the program will not be worth your time, money, and energy.

THANKS FOR READING!

What did you think of, **Understanding Obesity: A New Hope For Weight Loss and Escaping Food Addiction**

I know you could have picked any number of books to read, but you picked this book and for that I am extremely grateful.

I hope that it added at value and quality to your everyday life. If so, it would be really nice if you could share this book with your friends and family by posting to Facebook and Twitter.

If you enjoyed this book and found some benefit in reading this, I'd like to hear from you and hope that you could take some time to post a review. Your feedback and support will help this author to greatly improve his writing craft for future projects and make this book even better.

I want you, the reader, to know that your review is very important and so, if you'd like to leave a review, all you have to do is click here and away you go. I wish you all the best in your future success!

Thank you and good luck!

Madison Fuller

Claim This Now

Autoimmune Healing Transform Your Health, Reduce Inflammation, Heal the Immune System and Start Living Healthy

Do you have an overall sense of not feeling your best, but it has been going on so long that it's actually normal to you?

If you answered yes to any of these question, you may have an autoimmune disease.

Autoimmune diseases are one of the ten leading causes of death for women in all age groups and they affect nearly 25 million Americans.

In fact millions of people worldwide suffer from autoimmunity whether they know it or not.

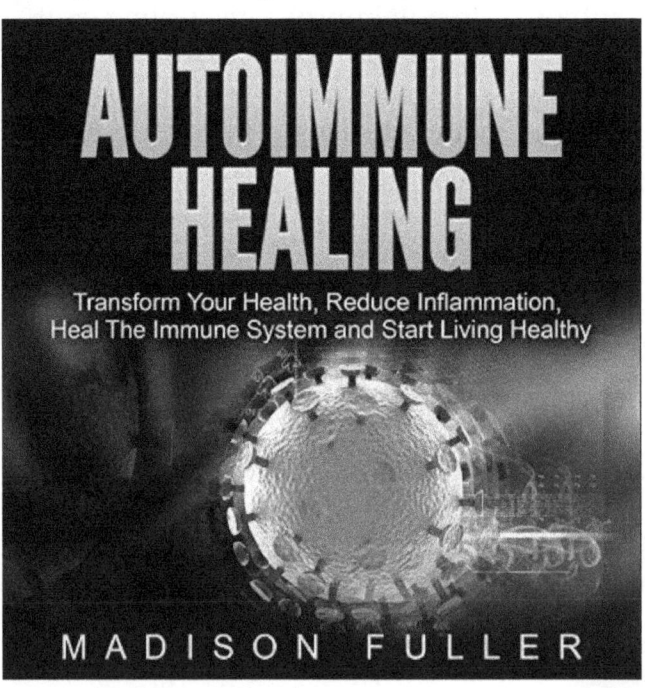

Want More?

Sign up to get the exclusive Madison Fuller e-newsletter, sent out a few times a week:

Sign Up

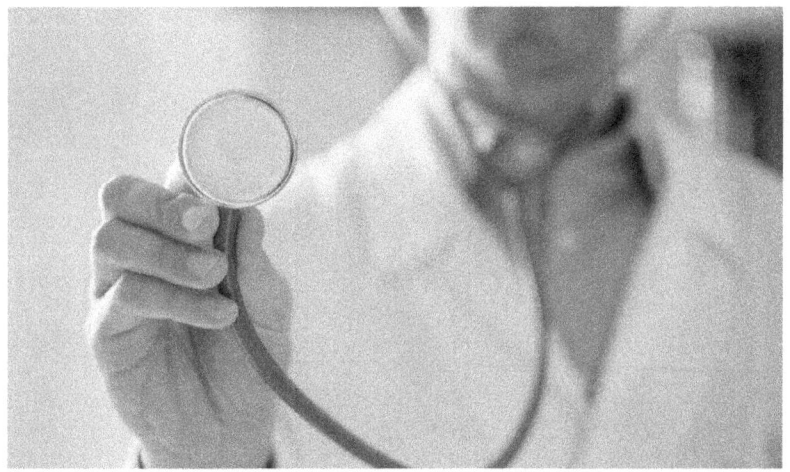

www.ingramcontent.com/pod-product-compliance
Lightning Source LLC
Chambersburg PA
CBHW030301030426
42336CB00009B/483